BY VEGANSOULFOOD.CO

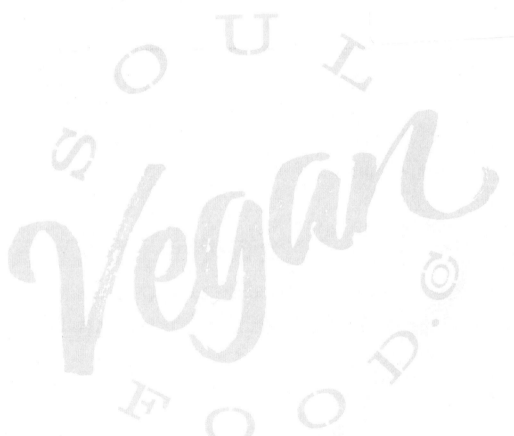

Vegan Soul Food is an idea that started from our facebook group: **Vegan Soul Food**.

Brooke Brimm, the founder of the group, had an idea to create a Vegan Soul Foodie group. A group where we encourage each other to create, enjoy, and share our love of plant-based food, without having to be 100% Vegan or plant-based.

All of our dishes and offerings are 100% plant-based, and shared with love and joy!

This guide is an extension of what we offer on our website and Social Media.

vegansoulfood.co

instagram.com/vegansoulfood.co

facebook.com/groups/vegansoulfood

A special acknowledgement to:

Sophie Williams and D. Monique Couch for assistance with family recipes.

Two members of the group have lovingly offered their recipes to add to this guide. Their names are by the recipes that they've offered.

We'd like to acknowledge:

Kalyn Hall Ewan, instagram.com/sweetpeppavegan
and
Latasha Cousar.

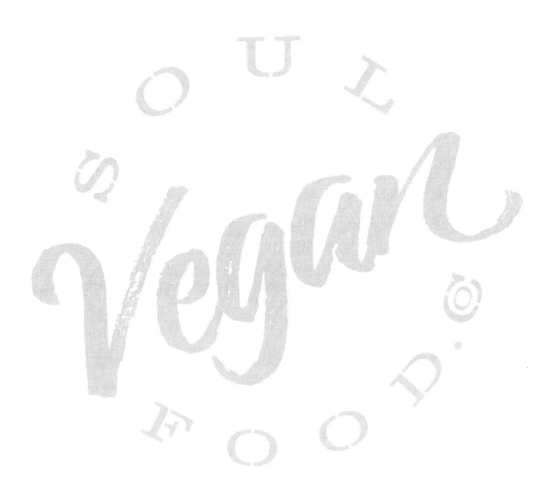

OUR STORY

Craig & Brooke Brimm have been on a plant-based journey since 1991. Since the early 1990's the Brimms have been either 100% plant-based, vegetarian, pescatarian, or raw plant-based.

Through the years they have gained an immense amount of knowledge about plant-based eating and cooking.

They want to share the best parts of being a plant-based foodie. No matter the food philosophy of friends, family, or guests, they can always expect to receive a delicious plant-based creation at the table of the Brimms.

Brooke, being the main plant-based chef in their home, has also extended her love of plant-based soul food to attendees at retreats that she hosts for women, brookebrimm.com/retreats.

Although the retreats are not 100% plant-based, all attendees get an opportunity to try out plant-based meal offerings, and often rave about how delicious they are, especially compared to the traditional soul food she prepares.

The Brimm children have joined in on the plant-based love by offering their assistance as administrators in the Facebook created by Brooke, Vegan Soul Food, which has a membership of over 70, 000 at the time of this printing.

This guide is all about how we do things at the holidays. Since all family members are not plant-based, some of the recipes have been "Veganized," so that you can enjoy a fully plant-based holiday.

APPETIZERS

Appetizers are a big part of our meals on the holidays. We don't usually serve breakfast, so we put out appetizers quite early.

They are out by the television as soon as the Thanksgiving Day parade begins, and they get refilled all they way up until the main meal is served.

Make your appetizers all about the veggies. Lay out a wide array of Crudités with items such as olives, roasted peppers, celery, carrots, pickles, cucumbers, and vegan cheese spreads, Miyoko's has a wide variety that you can find near you.

You can also find a wide variety of hummus and other vegan dips from Aldi, Whole Foods, Trader Joe's, and Farmer's markets.

RECIPES

Mushroom Bruschetta

1 pound of mixed mushrooms (white button, baby bella, Portabella, & shiitake. Use any blend that you like)

5 Tablespoons olive oil, plus 1 tablespoon

2 Tablespoon balsamic vinegar

1 Tablespoon fresh thyme leaves

1/4 cup Himalayan Pink Salt

Red crushed pepper

6 cloves of garlic, chopped

Instructions

1. Preheat oven to 400 degrees Fahrenheit.
2. De-stem any mushrooms with fibrous stems.
   Roughly chop mushrooms. Place all mushrooms in a large bowl and cover with water. Mix in the salt and leave mushrooms to soak for 15 minutes.
3. Remove mushrooms from the bowl and place them on a cookie sheet with a lip (the mushrooms will generate lots of liquid when cooking, you don't want it to spill out).
4. Coat the mushrooms with the 5 tablespoons olive oil, pepper, and ½ the chopped garlic.
5. Bake in oven for 15 minutes or until slightly brown and plump.
6. Remove mushrooms from oven, toss in remaining garlic, 1 tablespoon of olive oil and 2 tablespoons of balsamic vinegar, and fresh thyme leave.
7. Salt & red crushed pepper to taste.

Tomato Bruschetta

6 or 7 ripe tomatoes (about 1 1/2 pounds)

2 cloves garlic, minced (about 2 teaspoons)

1 Tablespoon extra virgin olive oil

1 teaspoon balsamic vinegar

6-8 fresh basil leaves, thinly sliced* or chopped

3/4 teaspoon sea salt, more or less to taste

1/2 teaspoon freshly ground black pepper, more or less to taste

Instructions

1. Remove the seeds tomatoes & chop them, small. Grate the fresh garlic on a microplane or use a garlic press. Cut the basil into Julienne your strips.
2. Place all items into a bowl together. Mix well and refrigerate for about 1 hour or longer to let the flavors meld together.
3. Serve all bruschetta on French bread, Italian bread, pita chips or tortilla chips.

DESSERTS

D esserts are a big part of the holidays. We live for them. The good news is that now we can enjoy sweet holiday drinks like plant-based egg nog, and flavored plant-based creamer for our coffees to have with our desserts.

There are also a plethora of choices for plant-based ice cream and whipped creams. With these amazing store-bought complements, it's a breeze to pair them with our Vegan Soul Food Desserts.

RECIPES

Mo-Mo's Sweet potato pie

3 Large sweet potatoes

1 stick vegan butter, softened

1/2 cup brown sugar, not packed

2 cups of white sugar

1 can of coconut condensed milk

5 tablespoons of Egg Replacement (Neat eggs, Just eggs, Follow Your Heart Eggs)

2 Teaspoon of nutmeg

1 Teaspoon ground cinnamon

1 Tablespoon lemon extract

1 Tablespoon Vanilla extract

1/4 teaspoon salt

1/4 teaspoon ginger

9 inch unbaked pie crust vegan

Instructions

1. Preheat oven to 350 degrees F. In a blender add hot sweet potatoes with butter until smooth. Add remaining ingredients except crust; blend well.
2. Pour into pie shell. Bake 40 minutes or until golden brown.
3. Cool. Garnish as desired.

Kalyn's Sweet potato pudding

6 cups grated sweet potato (about 1 and 1/2 large Japenese or
Boniata sweet potato)

3 cups brown sugar or cane sugar (I prefer brown sugar)

1 1/2 cups conrmeal

3 1/2 cups flour

1/4 cups vanilla

4 teaspoon almond extract

2 cans coconut milk

2 teaspoon baking powder

1 teaspoon nutmeg (I prefer grated)

1 teaspoon salt

2 teaspoon cinnamon

3 teaspoon rum (optional) I prefer Wray & Nephew White Rum

Vegan butter

Instructions

1. Preheat oven 325 degrees.
2. Wash and peel potatoes then add to food processor or grate them and place in a large mixing bowl.
3. Add sugar, flour, cornmeal, baking powder, and coconut milk.
4. Add nutmeg, cinnamon baking powder, rum, vanilla and almond extract, mix well.
5. Grease large glass baking dish with butter and pour in mixture.
6. Bake at 325 degrees for 1hour 30 min minutes or until knife comes out smooth.
7. Let sit for at least an hour then cut into squares and serve.

Note: This dish can be made the night before.

Latasha's Easy Banana Chocolate Chip Bread

2-3 very ripe bananas (approximately 1 cup)

1/2 cup of vegan chocolate chips divided (I use the Enjoy Life Morsels Dark Chocolate)

1-2 heaping tablespoon of peanut butter

1/2-3/4 cup of flour (your choice)

1/2 teaspoon vanilla extract

3 tablespoon non-dairy milk

1/3 cup brown sugar

3/4 teaspoon cinnamon

1/2 teaspoon baking soda

1/4 teaspoon salt

Instructions
1. Preheat oven to 350F. Lightly grease an 8"x8" baking pan.
2. Mash ripe bananas in a mixing boil. Add brown sugar, non-dairy milk, and vanilla to bananas. Mix well.
3. Sift in flour, cinnamon, baking soda, and salt to banana mixture.
4. Next gently fold in 1/4 cup of chocolate chips reserving the other 1/4 cup for the top.
5. Pour mixture into greased pan and spread evenly. Mixture will be fairly thick but pourable.
6. Sprinkle on top the remaining chocolate chips.
7. Bake for 15 to 20 minutes or until brown and toothpick comes out clean.
8. Let cool for at least 10 minutes then cut and serve.

Notes
- I use small bread pans to make mini loaves and it comes out perfect.
- I also add chopped pecans sometimes for a little crunch and variety.
- Add enough flour so mixture is thicker than pancake batter but not stiff like a dough. It should still be wet and pour into baking dish.

BREAD

B reads are usually an after thought on our holiday meal table. We have bread out for our appetizers, and by the time we are ready to chow down for the main meal, bread is a forgotten thought.

If you are putting bread on your table remember to check the labels for ingredients that are not plant-based such as eggs, milk, whey, and lactic acid. If you are especially concerned about where your breads were prepared, check the bottom of the label for words like "made with milk."

There are vegan apps to help you with identifying whether the item you are buying is 100% plant-based or not. Just scan the barcode to find out. Here is one:

Is It Vegan?

There are lots of items like frozen croissants that are vegan and enjoyable. Aldi carries items like these. The important thing to know is that you can have bread. It just takes a bit of savvy to find the ones you want.

Vegan buttermilk biscuits

2 cups flour

1/2 teaspoon salt

4 teaspoons baking powder

1 tablespoon sugar

1/2 cup vegan butter

2/3 cup plant milk

1 tablespoon of apple cider vinegar

Instructions

1. Preheat oven to 425° F. Place apple cider vinegar inside of the 2/3 of plant milk set it aside.
2. Put flour, salt, baking powder, and sugar into a bowl and mix. Cut in the vegan butter until mixture resembles course meal or pebbles.
3. Add plant milk mixture all at once and stir until dough forms a ball around the fork.
4. Turn dough onto a lightly floured surface and knead 14 times.
5. Pat dough until 1/2" thick and cut with a biscuit cutter.
6. Spray two 8" cake pans and place the cut out biscuits into it so they touch. Bake 15 - 20 minutes or until golden. Serves 12.
7. If you would like to make drop biscuits instead, increase your plant milk to 1 cup. Instead of rolling out the dough and cutting it with a cutter, just drop the biscuits from an end of a large spoon.

SIDES

The holidays are about the sides. We pile them on, and enjoy every one of them. Many of the recipes in this section have been in my family for decades. I have "veganized" them to fit the plant-based lifestyle. My family usually rotates where we hold our celebrations. When they are held at my house, most of the recipes are "veganized" and no one notices the difference.

Other sides in the section have been added by **Vegan Soul Food** Facebook Group Members.

RECIPES

Sophie's Cranberry Sauce

1 1/2 cups sugar

1 small can crushed pineapple, drained

1 small apple with skin diced

1/2 cup rough chopped walnuts

1 cups water

1 (12-oz.) package fresh cranberries

2 teaspoons orange zest

Instructions

1. In a small saucepan over low heat, combine sugar and water until sugar dissolves.
2. Add cranberries and cook until they burst, 12 minutes.
3. Mash the cranberries in saucepan.
4. Fold in orange zest, apples, walnuts & drained pineapple.
5. Add to mold. Refrigerate for 4 hours.
   Serves 10.

Soul food Vegan Greens

1/4 cup extra virgin olive oil

5 tablespoons vegan butter

1 large onion, minced

5 cloves garlic, minced

(Use a mix of two of your favorite greens here. We are using kale & mustard)

1 pound kale greens, chopped

1 pound mustard greens

2 tablespoons of mushroom seasoning

2 large tomatoes, chopped

5 mini sweet peppers, minced

2 jalapeños seeded & deveined

3 celery stalks minced

2 shallots chopped

Salt and freshly ground black pepper

Instructions

1. Mince all veggies except greens in a food processor.
2. Roughly chop greens. If you want very soft greens, remove the green stems.
3. Save them for juicing or a smoothie later.
4. Take the processed veggies and place into a stock pot or pressure cooker with butter & olive oil. Sauté on medium heat.
5. Slowly add in roughly chopped greens. Cover the greens with sautéed veggies. Liquid will start to form on the bottom. Slowly add in more greens & keep stirring. Add salt to allow more water to draw out of the veggies.

   Cover with lid and cook on low pressure for 12 minutes. Release pressure and serve.

   Serves 8.

CHECK OUT HOW THESE GREENS WERE MADE ON OUR IGTV.

instagram.com/vegansoulfood.com

Sophie's Garlic string (green) beans

2 pounds fresh string beans, trimmed

5 tablespoons olive oil

1 stick of vegan butter or margarine

10 cloves of chopped garlic

1/2 teaspoon Himalayan pink salt

1/4 teaspoon ground black pepper

Instructions

1. Steam green beans for 3 minutes.
2. Remove from heat & let cool or rinse with cool water. It depends on how bright green & crunchy you want your green beans. Cool water will keep them bright green.
3. Heat a large skillet over medium heat. Add the olive oil, margarine, garlic.
4. Once butter is melted, add string beans and stir. Add the salt and pepper, and continue to stir.
5. Cover string beans thoroughly. Serve. Cook 5 minutes longer if you want very tender beans.
   Serves 8.

Kalyn's Vegan Broccoli and Cheese Casserole

2 cups quinoa cooked

1 cup chopped broccoli

1 cup oat milk

Seasonings - garlic powder, onion powder, vegetable seasoning, pepper and salt

1 slice vegan gouda or cheddar cheese

1/4 cup vegan cheddar shreds

1/4 cup cashew cream

1/2 pack Ritz crackers crushed

Instructions

1. Make a roux with 1 tablespoon flour and vegan butter.
2. Add oat milk gradually stirring as sauce thickens, mix in vegan cheese slices, cashew cream, seasonings and chopped broccoli stiring until broccoli is cooked and cheeses is fully melted (add more oat milk as needed if too thick).
3. Stir in cooked quino and cheese shreds.
4. Top with crushed Ritz crackers and small pieces of butter.
   Bake at 350 for 30 - 45 min and serve.
   Serves 8.

New Orleans Vegan Dirty Rice

1 bag of vegan crumbles/burger, store bought

3 tablespoons Extra virgin olive oil,

1 large onion, finely diced

3 cloves garlic, minced

1 celery stalk, chopped

1/2 cup of mixed sweet bell peppers (I use mini-mixed sweet peppers)

1 Jalapeño chopped, de-seeded, & de-veined.

3 tablespoons Creole seasoning

1 tablespoon of Mushroom seasoning

1 cup water

3 cups parboiled brown rice, cooked

salt, to taste

scallion, chopped for garnish

Instructions
1. Sauté' vegan crumbles, set aside.
2. Heat oil in a large skillet on medium-high heat, add onion, garlic, celery, sweet peppers and cook until fragrant and soft, about 3 minutes.
3. Add Creole seasoning, mushroom seasoning and water. Bring to a boil. Cook for 3 minutes.
4. Stir in the vegan crumbles, rice, salt to taste and scallion. Cook until heated through, about 1 - 3 minutes or until liquid is evaporated.
   Serves 6.

Arroz con Gandules (Rice and Pigeon Peas)

Sofrito

3 cloves garlic

1 cup white onion

4 medium scallions

1/2 cup cilantro or culandro

1/2 cup sweet bell pepper (red, yellow, or orange)

1 medium tomato

1 tablespoon oil

1 15 oz can pigeon peas or gandules, drained or 2 cups of pigeon peas which have been pressured cooked.

2 cups of uncooked parboiled brown rice

3 cups water

1 tablespoon of mushroom seasoning

1 packet of Sazon

Salt to taste

Instructions

1. Chop all sofrito items in a food processor or chopper.
   In a heavy pot with a lid, heat oil on medium, add sofrito cook for three
2. minutes.
3. Add tomato and salt cook another minute. Stir in rice and blend well.
   Add Gandules (pigeon peas), water, mushroom seasoning, sazon, taste liquid
4. for flavor.
5. Mix well. Add salt to taste.
   Reduce flame to medium-low and let water boil down until it is
6. completely absorbed.
   Once there is just a bit of water in the pot, set flame to lowest setting and
7. cover for 20 minutes without stirring or lifting the lid.
   The steam will cook the rice.

Black-eyed peas and rice

1/4 cup olive oil

4 tablespoons of vegan butter

1 large onion, chopped

4 stalks of celery, chopped

6 cloves fresh garlic, minced

1/2 pound dried black-eyed peas if using Instant Pot, otherwise use 3 cups cooked or 2 15-ounce cans low- or no-sodium beans

1/2 cup uncooked parboiled brown rice

1 15-ounce can fire-roasted diced tomatoes

6 cups water

3 tablespoons of mushroom seasoning

1 tablespoon of granulated garlic

1 tablespoon of onion powder

2 whole bay leaves

1/2 of jalapeño seeded and deveined.

3 teaspoons Himalayan Pink Salt

1/2 teaspoon smoke paprika

Pressure cooker / Instant Pot Directions:

1. Sauté on medium heat, add onion and celery until translucent. Add the garlic and bay leaves and stir for 1-2 minutes.
2. Add the rest of the ingredients to the pot. Cover ingredients with water do not fill past the overfill line in the pot. Close the lid. Once the pot reaches pressure, cook for 25 minutes. Release the lid after 25 minutes. Stir and serve.

Stovetop Directions

1. In a large soup pot over medium high heat, water saute onion and celery until just becoming translucent. Add the garlic and rosemary and saute for 1-2 minutes or until garlic is fragrant, making sure not to burn garlic, adding 1-2 tablespoons water at a time, if necessary.
2. Add the rest of the items to the pot, stir to combine and bring to boil. Cover and lower heat to simmer for 30-45 minutes, stirring occasionally.

Latasha's Black-eyed Peas

1 pound (1 package) of dried black-eyed peas

1 onion sliced

1 teaspoon garlic powder

1 teaspoon onion powder

1 teaspoon smoked paprika

Vegetable broth or water

Salt and pepper to taste

1/2 of 12 oz jar prepared Sofrito or (Blend cilantro, onion, garlic, jalapeño, and Olive oil

Cholula Hot Sauce (to taste)

Sugar

Instructions

2. Soak peas overnight. Drain and rinse well before cooking.

3. In a deep pan or pot heat up 1 tablespoon of olive oil and sauté onion slices until soft.

4. Once onions are soft and drained and rinsed peas to pot.

5. Pour in vegetable broth or water until peas are covered.

6. Add in spices to pot. (I add salt later in the cooking process.)

7. Add in half a jar of Goya Sofrito and Cholula hot sauce. More or less can be added depending on taste.

Cook peas until tender and serve with your favorite vegan cornbread.

Carrot souffle

1 pound carrots, coarsely chopped

1/2 cup plant butter or margarine

1 teaspoon vanilla extract

3 tablespoons of vegan egg replacement

3 tablespoons all-purpose flour

1 teaspoon baking powder

1/2 teaspoon salt

3/4 cup white sugar

Instructions

1. Preheat oven to 350 degrees F (175 degrees C). Lightly oiled a 2 quart casserole dish.

2. Add peeled carrots to salted boiling water, and cook until tender, 15 to 20 minutes. Add carrots, margarine, vanilla extract and egg replacement, flour, baking powder, salt and sugar into a blender or food processor. Blend until smooth. Place mixture into prepared casserole dish. Bake for 45 minutes. **Serves 6.**

Kalyn's Potato, Pumpkin and Chickpea Curry

3 russet potatoes cut into large blocks

1/2 of a large calabaza squash or butternut squash cut into 2inch blocks

1 can Garbanzo beans (chick peas)

2 tblsp curry powder (I use Easispice, Blue Mountain or Chief brands)

2 garlic cloves chopped

1 onion chopped

1/4 c scallions chopped

3 sprigs thyme

1 teaspoon ginger paste

1 teaspoon green seasoning (I use Chief)

1/2 teaspoon of each: allspice powder, garlic powder, onion powder
and black pepper

1 can coconut milk

2 cans water

1 teaspoon salt

3 tablespoon vegetable oil

1 Scotch bonnet pepper (optional)

Instructions

1. In a large pot, mix curry powder with about 4 teaspoons water to make paste.
2. Add oil to pot let it warm up then add curry water paste and stir around.
3. Add and cook garlic, onion, scallions, ginger, green seasoning for 5min.
4. Add potato, chickpeas and squash.
5. Add can coconut milk, 2 can water which should be enough water to cover the veggies and dry seasonings, bring to boil.
6. Cover pot with lid and cook down on medium heat for 60 min stirring constantly and seasoning as needed, being sure not to let veggies burn at the bottom (add more water if needed).
7. Cook until you have a thick consistency and all large veggies are so soft they break apart.
   Serves 6.

Sophie's Candied Yams

3 pounds sweet potatoes

3 tablespoons of vegan butter or margarine

1/4 cup maple syrup

1/3 cup packed brown sugar

1 teaspoon cinnamon

1/4 teaspoon nutmeg

2 teaspoons lemon extract

2 teaspoons vanilla extract

Instructions

1. Scrub sweet potatoes with skin on. Steam or boil sweet potato with skin on until tender outside, but firm inside. Let cool, and peel skin off potatoes. Cut potatoes lengthwise into 2 - 3 pieces. Heat large cast iron skillet. Add butter, syrup, brown sugar, cinnamon, nutmeg, & extract to pan.

2. Once the mixture comes to a gentle bubble, add in sweet potatoes. Gently Coat sweet potatoes with heat on low for 10 mins.

   Serves 8.

Mo-Mo's Potato Salad

5 pounds Yukon Gold potatoes or Klondike Goldust potatoes

2 cups vegan mayo

1/2 cup sweet pickle relish

2 tablespoons yellow mustard

1 tablespoon of cayenne paper

1/4 teaspoon black salt (gives you the eggy flavor)

1 celery stalk, minced

1 medium sweet onion or red onion, minced

1 tablespoon fresh chopped dill

2 tablespoons of onion powder

1/2 tablespoon of adobe

1 teaspoon black pepper.

1/2 teaspoon Himalayan pink salt

1 tablespoon of salt to cook potatoes

Instructions

1. Scrub potatoes. Place whole potatoes in a large stock pot. Fill the pot with cold water until it is 1 inch over the top of the potatoes. Set the pot over high heat and bring to a boil. Once boiling, add 1 tablespoon salt and cook the potatoes until fork tender, about 15 minutes.

2. In a large bowl mix the vegan mayo, sweet pickle relish including juices, mustard. Stir until smooth. Then chop the celery, onions, and dill.

3. Once the potatoes are very tender, drain off all the water. Remove the loose peels and chop the potatoes into 1/2-inch chunks. They will be crumbly. Place the potatoes in a large bowl. Then stir in the celery, onions, and dill. After well mixed, place the mayo dressing into the bowl. Taste, then black, pink salt, and pepper as needed. Garnish with fresh dill and paprika.

4. Cover the potato salad and refrigerate for at least 4 hours. If you have time to make it ahead. Keep refrigerated in an airtight container for up to one week. **Serves 10.**

Garlic Mashed Potatoes

1 head of garlic

1 tablespoon extra virgin olive oil

2 pounds Yukon Gold potatoes

Salt to taste

Pepper to taste

1/3 cup vegan cream cheese

1/4 cup vegan butter

1/4 unsweetened vegan milk

Instructions

1. Preheat the oven to 425°
2. Cut off the stem end of the garlic head so that the cloves are exposed. Leave the head intact.
3. Drizzle olive oil over the garlic heads, salt lightly, and wrap in aluminum foil.
4. Bake at 425°F for 20 minutes, or until the cloves feel soft to the touch and are beginning to brown. Let cool.
5. Scrub potatoes with skins on. Cut into large pieces. Steam with skin on for 25 minutes or until potato is very tender.
6. Place the hot potatoes with all other ingredients except for garlic into a metal bowl or dutch oven. Squeeze garlic out of the skin into the potato mixture. Mash with a potato masher, mix with a mixer, or blend with a stick blender until the mixture is smooth. Season with salt & pepper.
Serves 8.

Vegan Cornbread Dressing

1 stick vegan butter

1 small sweet onion, chopped

4 stalks celery, chopped

1/2 cup fresh parsley, finely chopped,

3 small carrots grated

1/2 teaspoon dried sage

1/2 poultry seasoning

1/2 teaspoon dried thyme

1/2 teaspoon salt

2 1/2 cups water

2 tablespoons mushroom seasoning

3 cups prepared cornbread cut into small cubes. (vegetarian jiffy will work)

1 cup of shredded bread (white, wheat, rye, any kind you want is fine)

Instructions

1. Preheat oven to 350 degrees Fahrenheit.
2. Sauté veggies and stick of butter in a saucepan on medium low until softened and translucent. Add half the herb seasoning to the veggies. Add all of the mushroom seasoning to the veggies. Pour 2 1/2 cups water into the sauté mixture. Bring a simmer.
3. Mix the prepared cornbread and the shredded bread thoroughly. Pour the veggie mixture over the bread mixture. Mix well. Bake at 350 for 40 minutes or until browned on top.
   Serves 6.

Kalyn's Vegan Mac and Cheese

16 oz box macaroni noodles

2-3 packs Violife cheddar shreds

2 slices Follow your heart gouda cut into smaller pieces

1 violofe epic mature white cheddar block shredded

Seasonings: Garlic powder, Onion powder, Salt, Pepper, veggie seasoning

1/2 teaspoon tumeric for color

2 teaspoon Nutritional yeast

1/2 cup plain cashew cream (I use Forager)

4-5 cups Oat milk

Vegan butter

Instructions

1. Preheat oven to 350. Make roux with 2 tablespoon flour and 2 tblsp vegan butter. Cook noodles according to package, drain them and set aside.

2. Add oat milk gradually whisking out lumps to make a smooth sauce on low-medium heat (do not let sauce boil).

3. Stir in cashew cream, then add 2 slices of cheese, and half the pack cheddar shreds to the sauce, let melt. Add seasonings to your taste and stir until smooth. (You'll need about 4 cups of sauce to cover the noodles)

4. Add noodles to baking dish. Cover noodles in sauce and mix in half a pack shredded cheese and half cheddar block shreds. You can add more salt and pepper here if needed.

5. Add remaining white cheddar block shreds and enough cheddar shreds to cover the top.

6. Cover with foil and bake for 1 hour (Take foil off and bake uncovered for last 15 min watching closely).
   Serves 8.

Butternut Squash Mac n' Cheese

4 1/2 cups of cashew milk

1/2 cup of soaked raws cashew

3 tablespoons Yellow mustard

2 teaspoons smoked paprika

10 garlic cloves

1 ounce Himalayan pink salt

2 cups of nutritional yeast

2 cups of butternut squash puree

1 1/2 cups of vegetable oil

1 pound box of elbow macaroni

Instructions

1. Boil the noodles according to package instructions, drain & set aside. Blend all ingredients except the macaroni noodles. Pour blended mixture over the noodles and mix well. Place macaroni mixture into a large baking dish.
2. Bake for 45 mins at 350 degrees Fahrenheit.
   Serves 8.

Kalyn's Onion Gravy

1 onion chopped finely

1 tablespoon chopped scallion

1 celery stalk chopped finely

3 garlic cloves chopped finely

4 teaspoon flour

4 teaspoon vegan butter

1 tablespoon liquid aminos

1/2 teaspoon browning for color

1/2 teaspoon each - Onion powder, Garlic powder, Onion herb seasoning, Ground sage, cracked black pepper

1 tblsp salt

2 sprigs fresh thyme

2 bay leaf

32 oz carton veggie stock

Olive Oil

Salt to taste.

Instructions

1. Add 1 tblsp olive oil to pot and chopped veggies, cook for 3 min then remove veggies and set aside.
2. Add butter flour to make a roux cooking on low heat whisking until smooth
3. Return veggies and slowly add stock stirring constantly.
4. Add seasonings, bay leaf thyme, browning and aminos.
5. Let cook for 25 min on medium heat until desired thickness, seasoning to your taste as needed (use a cornstarch slurry to thicken if you needed).
6. Remove bay leaf and thyme. Strain out veggie bits.

Note: This can be made the night before.

Mushroom Gravy

1 Stick of vegan butter

3 cups thinly sliced baby bella mushrooms or white button mushrooms

1/2 cup finely minced onion

3 cloves garlic, minced

3 tablespoons all-purpose flour

2 tablespoons of mushroom seasoning

24 -32 ounces of water

salt and pepper to taste

Instructions

1. Sauté mushrooms, garlic, onion in butter on medium heat in a large skillet. Add flour, mushroom seasoning to 16 ounces of water. Stir into a slurry (a thickened water and flour mixture). Add the slurry to the sautéed veggies. Whisk together until smooth. Lower the heat. If the gravy gets too thick, add more water slowly until desired consistency. You may not use all 32 ounces. You may need a bit more water.
    Serves 8.

MAIN DISHES

W̲e may not eat a turkey or ham, but the main dish is a big deal for plant-eaters too. The following recipes are winners. When shopping for various mushrooms and canned jackfruit be sure to check out Asian farmer's markets.

RECIPES

Faux Dark Meat Un-Turkey

3 Large King Oyster Mushrooms

1 Large Portabella mushroom cap

7 Shitake Mushrooms, de-stemmed

2 tablespoon mushroom seasoning or Un-chicken seasoning

2 cloves of garlic, minced

1 large shallot chopped finely

1 teaspoon marjoram

1 teaspoon chervil

1 teaspoon basil

1 teaspoon ground rosemary

4 teaspoons ground sage

1 teaspoon ground thyme

1 tablespoon granulated garlic

1 teaspoon ground bay leaves

4 tablespoon extra virgin olive oil

1 1/2 cup of water

3 tablespoons flour

salt & pepper to taste

Instructions

1. Slice the portabella & Shiitake mushroom caps thinly, Shred the king oyster mushroom with a fork. Set aside. In an instant pot (electric pressure cooker) or pressure cooker, sauté shallots, garlic, mushrooms, seasonings, and herbs in olive oil for 2 minutes.

2. Pour in 1/2 cup of water into the mixture and place the lid on the pressure cooker. Cook on medium heat if using a stove pressure cooker. Cook on high, if using the instant pot (electric pressure cooker). Cook for 14 minutes. Bring the pressure down & open the lid. Mix 1 cup of water and 3 tablespoons together. Pour this mixture (slurry) into the mushrooms in the instant pot. Stir and allow mixture to thicken into a gravy mixture. Serve over mashed potatoes or brown rice.

Serves 8.

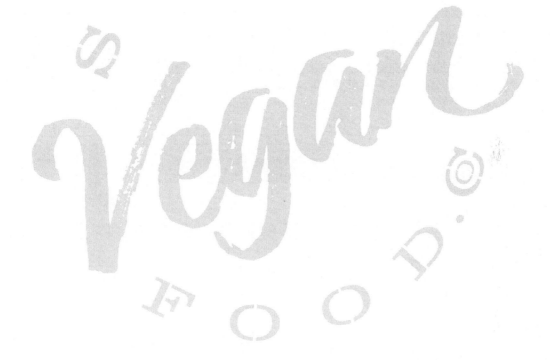

Chicken Fried Oyster Mushrooms

Wet Batter

1 cup all purpose flour

1 cup water more or less

1 teaspoon onion powder

1 teaspoon garlic powder

1 teaspoon sea salt

1 teaspoon of cajun or creole seasoning

1 teaspoon of mushroom seasoning

Dry Batter

1 cup flour

1 teaspoon onion powder

1 teaspoon garlic powder

1 teaspoon smoked paprika

1 teaspoon cajun or creole seasoning

1 teaspoon of dried parsley

32 ounce vegetable oil more or less for frying

1 package oyster mushrooms. Most Asian markets sell them

Instructions

1. Lightly wash your oyster mushrooms and drain them. Pull apart to desired pieces.
2. In a cast iron pan heat on medium high to high about 2-3 inches of oil.
3. Start making your wet batter. Batter should be pancake batter consistency to coat mushrooms; Set aside.
4. Place your dry batter into a large ziplock bag or paper bag.
5. Coat each oyster mushroom in the wet batter, then put them into the dry batter Ziploc bag shake and coat well.
6. Place each mushroom into the well heated pan of oil. It should sizzle when you put it in. Cook first side for about 2-3 minutes. Turn. When fully golden brown, take out and drain onto a paper towel or dish towel.

Serves 4.

Vegan Fried turkey cutlets

1 1/2 cup vital wheat gluten

Seasoned Wet mixture

1 cup of cooked pinto beans

1 shallot

1 medium onion

2 green onions

5 mini sweet peppers

2 teaspoons ground sage

1 teaspoon ground thyme

1 teaspoon ground rosemary

3 tablespoons granulated garlic

2 teaspoons onion powder

1 teaspoon basil

1 teaspoon marjoram

1 teaspoon chervil

3 tablespoons maple syrup

1 teaspoon creole seasoning

1 teaspoon grill seasoning

1 tablespoon steak sauce

2 tablespoons soy sauce or Liquid Aminos

1 tablespoon mushroom seasoning

2 Shredded king oyster mushrooms

1/2 can of green young jackfruit in water or brine

32 ounce vegetable oil more or less for frying

Wet Batter

1 cup all purpose flour

1 cup water more or less

1 teaspoon onion powder

1 teaspoon garlic powder

1 teaspoon sea salt

1 teaspoon of mushroom seasoning

Dry Batter

1 cup Panko bread crumbs

1 cup of flour

1 teaspoon onion powder

1 teaspoon garlic powder

1 teaspoon smoked paprika

1 teaspoon sage

1 teaspoon of dried parsley

Instructions

1. Shred the king oyster mushrooms with a fork. Break up the jackfruit. Set aside. Blend until smooth pinto beans and other ingredients for the seasoned wet mixture. Mix shredded jackfruit, mushrooms, vital wheat gluten and seasoned wet mixture in a bowl, save about 5 tablespoons of the seasoned wet mixture aside. Mix and knead for about 2-3 minutes or until mixture is thoroughly integrated. Cut 3 inch round piece of the seitan mixture and roll it with a rolling pin. Brush it with some seasoned wet mixture that you set aside. Place the flattened round in a piece of parchment paper and fold it up. Wrap in foil. Keep making packets of parchment and foil covered seitan cutlets. Place all in a double boiler or steamer. Steam for 30 minutes.

2. Start making your wet batter. Batter should be pancake batter consistency to coat mushrooms; Set aside. Place your dry batter into a large ziplock bag or paper bag.

3. Remove seitan flats from foil packets. It will be bigger in size.

4. In a cast iron pan heat on medium high to high about 2-3 inches of oil.

5. Coat each cutlet in the wet batter, then put them into the dry batter Ziploc bag shake and coat well.

6. Place each cutlet into the well heated pan of oil. It should sizzle when you put it in. Cook first side for about 2-3 minutes. Turn. When fully golden brown, take out and drain onto a paper towel or dish towel.

Serves 8.

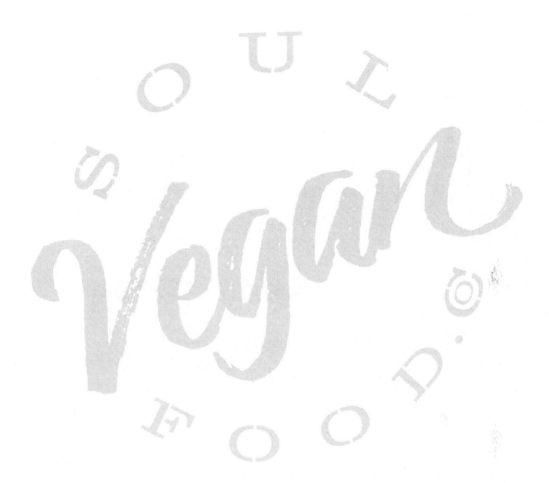

CHECK OUT HOW THE VEGAN FRIED TURKEY CUTLETS WERE MADE ON OUR IGTV.

instagram.com/vegansoulfood.com

Vegan Ribs

1 1/2 cup vital wheat gluten

Seasoned Wet mixture

1 cup of cooked pinto beans

1 shallot

1 medium onion

2 green onions

5 mini sweet peppers

2 teaspoons smoked paprika

3 tablespoons granulated garlic

2 teaspoons onion powder

2 teaspoons chili powder

3 tablespoons maple syrup

1 teaspoon creole seasoning

1 teaspoon grill seasoning

1 tablespoon steak sauce

2 tablespoons soy sauce or Liquid Aminos

1 tablespoon mushroom seasoning

2 Shredded king oyster mushrooms

1/2 can of green young jackfruit in water or brine

2 bottles of prepared barbecue sauce.

Instructions

1. Preheat oven to 300 degrees.
2. Shred the king oyster mushrooms with a fork. Break up the jackfruit. Set aside. Blend until smooth pinto beans and other ingredients for the seasoned wet mixture. Mix shredded jackfruit, mushrooms, vital wheat gluten and seasoned wet mixture in a bowl. Mix and knead for about 2-3 minutes or until mixture

is thoroughly integrated. Pour whole bottle of barbecue sauce into a shallow baking dish. Transfer vital wheat gluten mixture into the shallow dish and coat well. Turn over and continue to coat. It will be a bit messy. Place in the oven for 2 hours on 300 degrees. Baste it with its own sauce every 20 minutes. When sauce is caramelized, remove from oven & score seitan into squares or rectangles.

CHECK OUT HOW THE VEGAN RIBS WERE MADE ON OUR IGTV.

instagram.com/vegansoulfood.com

Printed in Great Britain
by Amazon